HEALTH BENEFITS OF VITAMIN B12

Unveiling the multi-purpose function of vitamin B12

(cobalamin)

BY

Dr. DOUGLAS JASON

DEDICATION

This book is committed to God All-powerful for the motivation to compose this extraordinary abundance of information. and likewise, to those who are having some deficiency traceable to vitaminB12.

ACKNOWLEDGEMENT

I truly value Dr. Katrina Kellogg(head of dietician departments, Shafi medical complex)for his help with the writeup of this incredible abundance of information. also to all staff members of Bebe clinic.

ABOUT THE AUTHOR

DR DOUGLAS JASON is a guaranteed dietician with huge excitement for helping people with continuing with a strong life through the use of good food sources, flavors, and spices.

INTRODUCTION

Vitamin B12 assumes a critical part in numerous parts of well-being and may uphold bone well-being, red platelet development, energy levels, and state of mind.

Eating a nutritious, balanced diet or taking an enhancement can assist with guaranteeing you're addressing your necessities.

Vitamin B12, otherwise called cobalamin, is a fundamental nutrient that your body needs yet can't create.

It's tracked down normally in creature items, yet additionally added to specific food varieties and accessible as an oral enhancement or infusion.

Vitamin B12 plays many parts in your body. It upholds the ordinary capability of your nerve cells and is required for red platelet development and DNA blend

For most grown-ups, the suggested dietary stipend (RDA) is 2.4 micrograms (mcg), however, it's higher for individuals who are pregnant or breastfeeding.

Vitamin B12 might help your body in amazing ways, for example, by supporting your energy, working on your memory, and helping prevent coronary illness.

Thus in this book, I will show you the medical advantages of vitamin B12, which are completely based on science.

TABLE OF CONTENT

DEDICATION

ACKNOWLEDGMENT

ABOUT THE AUTHOR

INTRODUCTION

CHAPTER 9

SUPPORT HEALTHY HAIR, SKIN, AND NAILS.

CONCLUSION

CHAPTER 1

AIDS RED BLOOD CELL FORMATION AND PREVENT ANEMIA

Vitamin B12 assumes a crucial part in assisting your body with creating red platelets.

Low vitamin B12 levels can also cause a decrease in red platelet arrangement and keep them from growing appropriately.

Solid red platelets are little and round, though they become bigger and ordinarily oval in instances of lack of vitamin B12.

Because of this bigger and unpredictable shape, the red platelets can't move from the bone marrow into the circulatory system at a suitable rate, causing megaloblastic weakness.

At the point when you have sickliness, your body needs more red platelets to move oxygen to your fundamental organs. This can cause side effects like exhaustion and shortcoming.

VITAL TIP

Vitamin B12 is engaged with red platelet arrangement. At the point when vitamin B12 levels are too low, the development of red platelets is adjusted, causing megaloblastic paleness.

CHAPTER 2

PREVENT MAJOR BIRTH DEFECTS

Satisfactory vitamin B12 levels are essential to a solid pregnancy.

Concentrates on showing that a baby's mind and sensory system require adequate B12 levels from the mother to appropriately create.

Lack of vitamin B12 in the early phases of pregnancy might expand the gamble of birth absconds, for example, brain tube deserts.

Moreover, maternal vitamin B12 inadequacy might add to untimely birth or premature delivery.

One more established investigation discovered that females with vitamin B12 levels lower than 250 milligrams for each deciliter (mg/dL) were multiple times bound to bring forth a kid with birth surrenders, contrasted with those with satisfactory levels.

For females with a lack of vitamin B12 and levels under 150 mg/dL the gamble was multiple times higher, contrasted with those with levels over 400 mg/dL.

VITAL TIP

Proper vitamin B12 levels are critical to a sound pregnancy.

They're significant for the avoidance of mind and spinal rope birth abandons.

CHAPTER 3

SUPPORT BONE HEALTH AND PREVENT OSTEOPOROSIS.

Keeping up with sufficient vitamin B12 levels might uphold your bone well-being.

One concentrate in 110 individuals with celiac illness observed that low degrees of vitamin B12 were connected to diminished bone mineral thickness in the femur and hips in guys.

Bones with diminished mineral thickness can become sensitive and delicate over the long haul, prompting an expanded gamble of osteoporosis.

A few different examinations have likewise shown a connection between low vitamin B12 levels and unfortunate bone well-being and osteoporosis or crack gamble.

Be that as it may, different investigations have turned up mixed results on the impacts of vitamin B12 on bone well-being, so more examination is required.

VITAL TIP

Vitamin B12 might assume an imperative part of our-bone well-being. Low blood levels of this nutrient have been related to an expanded gamble of osteoporosis and diminished bone thickness.

CHAPTER 4

REDUCE YOUR RISK OF MACULAR DEGENERATION

Macular degeneration is an eye illness that influences your focal vision.

Keeping up with sufficient degrees of vitamin B12 might assist with forestalling the gamble old enough related to macular degeneration.

Specialists accept that enhancing with vitamin B12 might bring down degrees of homocysteine, a kind of amino corrosive that is tracked down in your circulation system

Raised homocysteine levels have been related to an expanded gamble old enough related macular degeneration.

A recent report including around 5,000 females matured 40 or more established inferred that enhancing with vitamin B12, alongside folic corrosive and vitamin B6, may lessen this gamble.

The gathering getting these enhancements for quite a long time had fewer instances of macular degeneration, contrasted with the fake treatment bunch.

The gamble of fostering any type of condition was 34% lower, while it was 41% lower for additional serious sorts.

Eventually, further examinations are expected to completely comprehend vitamin B12's part in advancing vision well-being and forestalling macular degeneration.

VITAL TIP

Keeping up with satisfactory degrees of vitamin B12 diminishes homocysteine levels in your blood. This might assist with forestalling the advancement of old enough related macular degeneration.

CHAPTER 5

IMPROVE MOOD AND SYMPTOMS OF DEPRESSION.

Vitamin B12 might work on your temperament.

The impact of vitamin B12 on temperament isn't yet completely comprehended.

Nonetheless, this nutrient assumes an essential part in blending and processing serotonin, a compound liable for managing mindset.

Consequently, vitamin B12 inadequacy might prompt diminished serotonin creation, which can cause a discouraged state of mind.

One more seasoned concentrate on individuals with sadness and vitamin B12 levels on the low side of typical found that the people who got the two antidepressants and vitamin B12 were bound to show worked on burdensome side effects, contrasted with those treated with antidepressants alone.

In a huge survey, specialists found that lack of vitamin B12 was related to a higher gamble of misery, however just in more established females.

However vitamin B12 enhancements might assist with further developing mindset and sadness in individuals with a lack, research doesn't at present recommend that they have a similar impact in those with ordinary B12 levels.

Vitamin B12 is required for the development of serotonin, a compound liable for managing the state of mind. Vitamin B12 enhancements might assist with further developing temperament in individuals with a lack of current.

CHAPTER 6

PREVENT LOSS OF NEURONS IN THE BRAIN

Lack of vitamin B12 has been related to cognitive decline, particularly in more seasoned grown-ups.

The nutrient assumes a part in forestalling cerebrum decay, which is the deficiency of neurons in the mind and is frequently connected with cognitive decline or dementia.

One concentrate in individuals with beginning-phase dementia showed that a blend of vitamin B12 and omega-3 unsaturated fat enhancements eased back cognitive deterioration.

Another investigation discovered that even vitamin B12 levels on the low side of typical can add to unfortunate memory execution.

Nonetheless, different examinations show that vitamin B12 supplementation is probably insufficient for working on mental capability in those without a lack.

Subsequently, more exploration is expected to make sound ends on the impact of vitamin B12 supplements on memory and mental capability.

VITAL TIP

Vitamin B12 might assist with forestalling mind decay and cognitive decline.

More examination is expected to finish up if enhancing this nutrient can further develop memory in those without a lack.

CHAPTER 7

GIVES YOU AN ENERGY BOOST

Vitamin B12 supplements have for some time been promoted as the go-to item for a flood of energy.

All B nutrients assume a significant part in your body's energy creation, however, they aren't guaranteed to give energy themselves.

At present, there is no logical proof to propose that vitamin B12 enhancements can help energy in those with adequate levels of this nutrient.

Then again, if you're essentially lacking in vitamin B12, taking an enhancement or expanding your admission will probably further develop your energy level.

Truth be told, one of the most widely recognized early indications of a lack of vitamin B12 is weariness or absence of energy.

Vitamin B12 is associated with energy creation in your body.

Taking an enhancement might further develop your energy level, however, provided that you're lacking in this nutrient.

CHAPTER 8

IMPROVE HEART HEALTH BY DECREASING HOMOCYSTEINE

High blood levels of the amino corrosive homocysteine have been connected to an expanded gamble of coronary illness.

Assuming you're fundamentally lacking in vitamin B12, your homocysteine levels become raised.

Studies have shown that vitamin B12 helps decline homocysteine levels, which might lessen your gamble of coronary illness.

In any case, there is right now no logical proof to affirm that vitamin B12 supplements assist with forestalling coronary illness.

Consequently, further examination is expected to grasp the connection between vitamin B12 and heart well-being.

VITAL TIP

Vitamin B12 can also diminish blood homocysteine, a sort of amino corrosive that is related to an expanded gamble of coronary illness.

In any case, research doesn't as of now support the case that vitamin B12 diminishes this gamble.

CHAPTER 9

SUPPORT HEALTHY HAIR, SKIN, AND NAILS

Given vitamin B12's part in cell creation, satisfactory levels of this nutrient are expected to advance solid hair, skin, and nails.

Truth be told, low vitamin B12 levels can cause different dermatologic side effects, including hyperpigmentation, nail staining, hair changes, vitiligo (the deficiency of skin variety in patches), and rakish stomatitis (aggravated and broken mouth corners).

Enhancing with vitamin B12 has been displayed to work on dermatologic side effects in individuals with a B12 lack.

Nonetheless, it's hazy whether taking an enhancement anily affects skin, nail strength, or hair well-being on the off chance that you're very much fed and not lacking in this nutrient.

Solid vitamin B12 levels are significant for your hair, skin, and nails.

Be that as it may, taking an enhancement likely will not work on your well-being there for your levels are as of now adequate.

CONCLUSION

An expected 3% of grown-ups in the US lack vitamin B12, while around 26% have low to typical or fringe lacking levels.

Lack of vitamin B12 can happen in one of two ways. Either your eating regimen needs satisfaction measures of it or your body can't completely ingest it from the food you eat.

In any case, some individuals are bound to lack vitaminB12
They incorporate
more established grown-ups
individuals with gastrointestinal issues, like Crohn's sickness or celiac infection
the individuals who have had gastrointestinal medical procedures, for example, bariatric medical procedures or gut resection medical procedure
individuals on a severely vegetarian diet

the people who take metformin for glucose
control

those taking proton siphon inhibitors for
persistent indigestion

In numerous more established grown-ups,
the discharge of hydrochloric corrosive in
the stomach is diminished, causing a
decrease in the retention of vitamin B12.

Assuming your body experiences issues
retaining vitamin B12, your primary care
physician might prescribe intramuscular
infusions of B12 to build your levels.

Dynamic vitamin B12 is just tracked down
normally in creature items. While the facts
confirm that particular sorts of ocean growth
and matured food varieties contain vitamin
B12, it's ordinarily in its latent structure,
otherwise called pseudovitamin B12.

Even though some plant-based milk or
grains might have been sustained with
vitamin B12, vegetarians who eat less are in

many cases restricted in this nutrient, jeopardizing individuals of lack.

If you eat a very arranged, nutritious, and changed diet, forestalling a lack of vitamin B12 ought to be simple. Nonetheless, on the off chance that you imagine that you may be in danger, address a specialist.

Lack of vitamin B12 can most frequently be forestalled or settled with oral or intramuscular infusions.

Risk factors for lack of vitamin B12 incorporate a diminished capacity to retain this nutrient because of low hydrochloric corrosive discharge, certain drugs, or gastrointestinal illness and medical procedures.

Vegetarian individuals are likewise in danger since B12 is tracked down in creature items.

Vitamin B12 is a water-solvent nutrient that you should get through diet or enhancements.

It's liable for the majority of physical processes and may help your well-being in different ways, for example, by forestalling significant birth absconds, supporting bone wellbeing, further developing state of mind, and keeping up with sound skin and hair.

Helping sufficient vitamin B12 through your eating routine is urgent. Nonetheless, on the off chance that you battle to get enough or have a condition that influences retention, supplements are a basic method for expanding your B12 consumption.